Monthly Doodle Challenge

Doodle Notebook

January Doodle Challenge

1. Word of the Year
2. Goal/Resolution
3. Hot Chocolate
4. Self Portrait
5. Snow Scene
6. What You Are Grateful For
7. Animal
8. Feeling
9. What Needs To Be Organized
10. What's New
11. What You Enjoy Eating
12. Maze
13. Your View Everyday
14. Chinese New Year Animal
15. Pair of Mittens
16. Winter Bird
17. Lamp
18. Draw With A Color
19. Evergreen Tree
20. Snow Scene With Water
21. Martin Luther King Jr.
22. Parade
23. Icicles
24. Reflection Of A Thought
25. Mountains
26. Stretch Yourself
27. Clear Mind
28. Comforting Heat
29. Vacation You Want To Take
30. Sunshine
31. Reflection On This Month

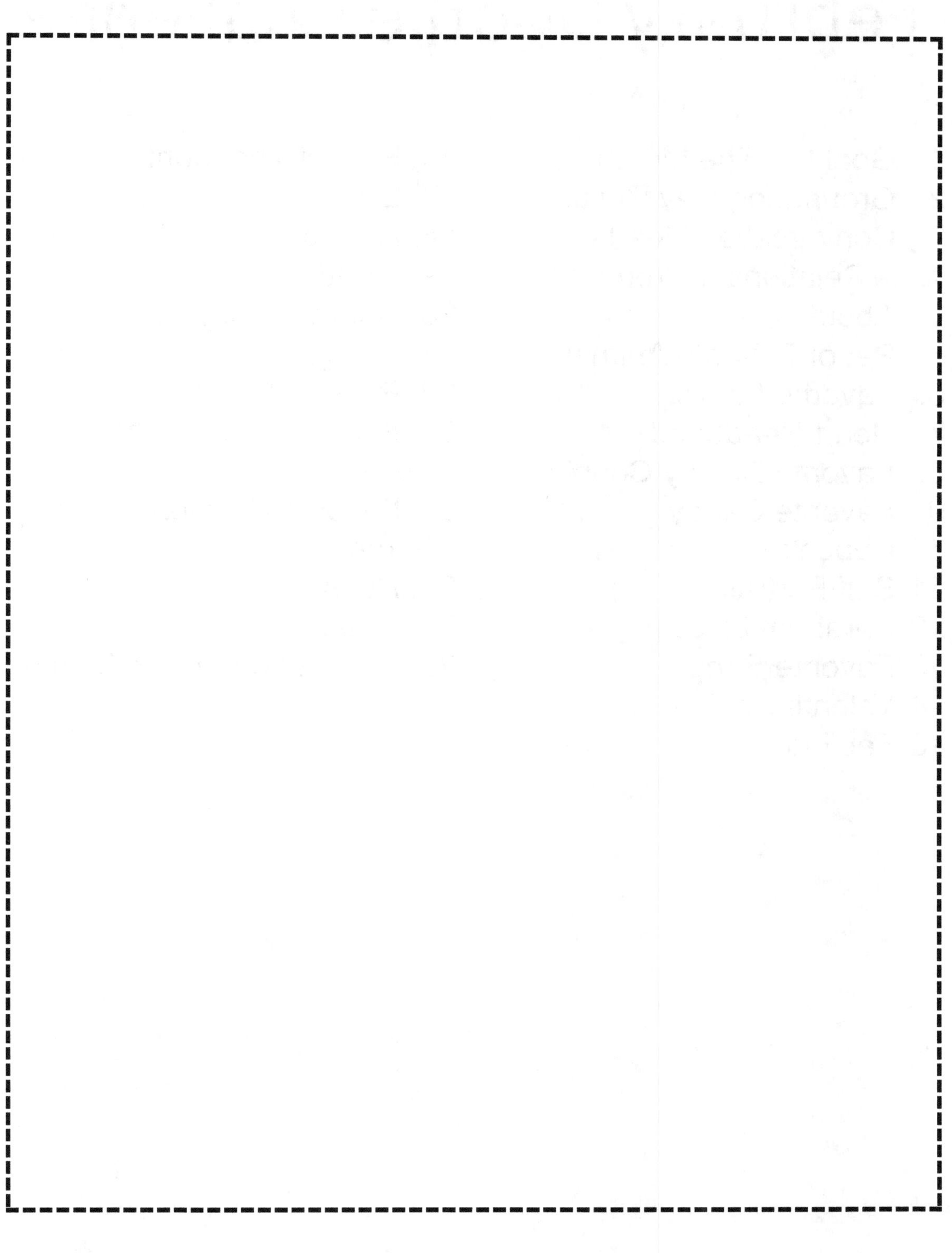

February Doodle Challenge

1. Goal For The Month
2. Groundhog Day Result
3. Conversation Hearts
4. A Relationship You Care About
5. Pet or Favorite Animal
6. Favorite Flower
7. Heart Headband
8. Favorite Disney Couple
9. Favorite Candy
10. Cupcake
11. Self Portrait
12. Abraham Lincoln
13. Favorite Song
14. Valentine's Day
15. Feeling
16. Bird Of The Month
17. Love
18. Hearts
19. Mandala
20. Happy Thoughts
21. Design
22. Peas In A Pod
23. Fashion
24. Art
25. Favorite Cartoon Character
26. Hugs
27. Wreath
28. Reflection For The Month

March Doodle Challenge

1. Goal For The Month
2. Shamrocks
3. Leprechaun
4. Pot of Gold
5. Mardi Gras
6. Faith
7. Rain
8. Swirl
9. Self Portrait
10. Feeling
11. Decision
12. Exercise/Fitness Activity You Do
13. Leaves
14. Shape
15. Ides of March
16. Favorite Crystal
17. St. Patrick's Day
18. Favorite Candle Smell
19. What's Going On In Space
20. Dream
21. What's Going On Today
22. Fun
23. Whale
24. Streetlight
25. Flower
26. A Song On The Radio
27. Word
28. Field Of Wildflowers
29. What's On Your Phone
30. Bookcase
31. Reflection For The Month

April Doodle Challenge

1. Goal For The Month
2. Bunny
3. Egg Hunt Scene
4. Colored & Designed Eggs
5. Daffodil
6. Dragonfly
7. Design
8. Flowering Tree
9. Instrument
10. Rain Boots & Umbrella
11. Feeling
12. Self Portrait
13. Rock
14. Activity You Enjoy
15. Daily Work
16. Unicorn
17. Frame
18. Raindrops
19. Color
20. World
21. Easter
22. Earth Day
23. Gratitude
24. Word
25. Food
26. Scene Outside
27. Learning
28. Mindfulness Drawing
29. Joy
30. Reflection For The Month

May Doodle Challenge

1. Goal For The Month
2. May's Flowers
3. Dog
4. Writing
5. Cinco de Mayo
6. Mandala
7. Design
8. Family
9. Hustle
10. School's Out
11. Where You Live
12. Mother's Day/Mom
13. Hero
14. Morning
15. Pasta
16. Boat
17. Pizza
18. Protection
19. Pizza
20. Favorite Décor
21. Diva
22. Sign
23. Fairy Wings
24. Llama
25. Circus
26. Smile
27. Memorial Day
28. Self Portrait
29. Border
30. Hands
31. Reflection For The Month

June Doodle Challenge

1. Goal For The Month
2. Father's Day/Dad
3. Planting
4. Healthy
5. Border Doodle
6. Route 66
7. Donut
8. Cuddles
9. Blessing
10. Flowers
11. Party
12. Think Positive
13. Fish
14. Favorite Summer Treat
15. Sunshine
16. Doodle Dangle
17. Wreath
18. Road Trip/Vacation
19. Cactus
20. Favorite Summer Food
21. Summer Solstice
22. Lighthouse
23. Leaves
24. Growing Season
25. Spirit Animal
26. Self Portrait
27. Sprinklers
28. Owl
29. Light Bulb
30. Reflection For The Month

July Doodle Challenge

1. Goal For The Month
2. Hot Dogs
3. Fireworks
4. 4th of July Celebration
5. Toucan
6. Summer Flower
7. Cat
8. Wreath
9. Self Portrait
10. Star Border
11. Heart Doodle
12. Letter Of Your 1st Name
13. Stripes
14. Beach Umbrella
15. Lightning Bugs
16. 16. Bicycle

17. Coffee
18. Crickets
19. Mandala
20. Daisy
21. Quilt Pattern
22. Watermelon
23. Flag
24. School Supplies
25. Sea Creature
26. Bees/Bee Hive
27. Camera
28. Hat
29. Circle Doodles
30. Kind Words
31. Reflection For The Month

August Doodle Challenge

1. Goal For The Month
2. Bird
3. Favorite Food
4. Fruits
5. Spirals
6. Moon
7. School
8. Surfboard
9. Beach
10. Dream Vacation
11. Favorite Drink
12. Exotic Animal
13. Favorite Quote
14. Dreamcatcher
15. August Weather Today
16. Mason Jars
17. Balloons
18. Wonder
19. Flower Box
20. Tulips
21. Butterfly
22. Root Beer Float
23. Fair/Festival
24. Relax
25. Popsicle
26. Pineapple
27. Sunshine
28. Ferris Wheel
29. Pool
30. Home
31. Reflection For The Month

September Doodle Challenge

1. Goal For The Month
2. Autumn
3. Mum Flowers
4. Hello Fall
5. Wreath
6. Acorn
7. Leaves
8. Bear Tracks
9. Favorite Soup
10. Teacup
11. Harvest
12. Self Portrait
13. Sky
14. Favorite Pie
15. Magical
17. Mushroom
18. Hedgehog
19. Sweater
20. Tent
21. Hot Drink
22. Leaf Dangles
23. Happy
24. State You Live In
25. Musical Notes
26. Hydrangea
27. Emoji Doodles
28. Planets
29. Divider Doodles
30. Clouds
31. Reflection For The Month

October Doodle Challenge

1. Goal For The Month
2. Spooky
3. Skeleton
4. Ghost
5. Pumpkin
6. Fall Weather
7. Spider Web
8. Mummy
9. Favorite Scary Story/Costume
10. Boo!
11. Hello October
12. Cupcake
13. Bat
14. Spider Web Border
15. Cat
16. Witch
17. Witches Brew
18. Frankenstein
19. Carved Pumpkin
20. Potion
21. Leaves Falling
22. Candy Corn
23. Candy Doodles
24. Favorite Costume
25. Fox
26. Wreath
27. Self Portrait
28. Trick Or Treat
29. Moon
30. Halloween
31. Reflection For The Month

November Doodle Challenge

1. Goal For The Month
2. Hello November
3. Deer
4. Football
5. Spirit
6. Warm Hugs
7. Mittens
8. Snow globe
9. Good Book
10. Cat Playing With Yarn
11. Turkey
12. Gratitude
13. Food
14. Table Setting
15. Family
16. Corn
17. Floral Doodle
18. Doodle Design
19. Cornucopia
20. Your Name
21. Wishing Tree
22. Turtle
23. Wreath
24. Maze
25. Drums
26. Surprise
27. Shopping 28. Thanksgiving
29. Travel
30. Reflection For The Month

December Doodle Challenge

1. Goal For The Month
2. Hello December
3. Christmas Lights
4. Warm Hat
5. Hot Drink
6. Fire in Fireplace
7. Reindeer
8. Ornament Dangles
9. Decorative Border
10. Stockings
11. Ornament
12. Tree
13. Snowflake
14. Gingerbread Man
15. Star Doodles
16. Dove
17. Peppermint Candy Cane
18. Holiday Border
19. Sled
20. Elf
21. Snow Globe Scene
22. Santa
23. Holiday Flower/Plant
24. Faith
25. Favorite Holiday
26. Sharing
27. Cookies
28. Mailbox
29. Wreath
30. Quote
31. Reflection For The Month

Prompt: ____

Doodle & Journal

Doodle & Bullet Journal

Doodle List

Doodle List

Monday

Tuesday

Wednesday

Thursday

Friday

Saturday

Sunday